Saffron Extract Weight Loss
Is It For All Overweight And Obese Persons?

I0426130

Jonas Lee

LEGAL NOTICE

The Publisher has strived to be as accurate and complete as possible in the creation of this publication, notwithstanding the fact that he does not warrant or represent at any time that the contents within are accurate due to new research data and findings.

In practical advice books, like anything else in life, there are no guarantees of absolute results made. Readers are cautioned to use their own judgment and discretion about their individual circumstances to act accordingly.

This book is not intended for use as a source of medical or treatment advice. All readers are advised to seek services of competent professionals in medical, nutrition, and health field.

Perceived slights of specific people or organizations are unintentional.

DISCLAIMER

While this guide is meant to provide you with the information you need to lose weight, it is highly recommend that you consult a physician before you begin taking any supplements, any form of physical activity or follow any of the suggestions in this book.

If you have any side effects as a result of the following information, consult a physician immediately. I am not a doctor, and this publication is provided for informational purposes only.

Table Of Contents

Chapter 1. Introduction

First of all, thank you for purchasing 'Saffron Extract Weight Loss: *Is It For All Overweight And Obese Persons?*'

Why Saffron Extract Weight Loss

As a person keenly interested in health and anything that influences the well-being of the body, I first came to know about Saffron Extract when I opened an email which linked to a Saffron Extract product in the market. As I read through the sales page of the product, I was drawn into it and inadvertently started to read up on any information I could find on this supplement.

Saffron Extract Supplement in the Limelight

Saffron extract has enjoyed the widespread publicity through Dr. Oz Show back in 2012. It is most well-known for its weight loss effects as many had witnessed on the Dr. Oz show. If you had been searching for an effective method for shedding some extra weight when the show was aired, you would likely be tempted to give it a try.

Is Saffron Extract Weight Loss Overhyped?

We must compliment Dr. Oz for his effort, other than being entertaining, to spread extensive information and knowledge on health products and health related issues. While Dr. Oz tried to cover as many grounds as possible, the valuable air time for a celebrity show can be restrictive. Therefore, an audience watching such a show could easily be drawn into the hype without understanding the ins and outs of a product. At times, this could be risky if one simply goes out to purchase and start consuming the product without knowing what are the limitations and risks of the substance.

While most people have heard about Saffron or Saffron Extract, but many are not certain how saffron extract works to produce weight loss effects in the body. The intention of this book is to provide information of saffron extract all in one place while attempting to bring a balanced view of this much publicized supplement.

As with any health product or supplement, we need to know its positive as well as negative impact on our body and health. It is my intention to share with my readers important information related to saffron and saffron extract. It is my hope that the reader will have sufficient information and knowledge to make an intelligent decision whether or not he or she should take the product.

Some answers and benefits in reading this Saffron Extract Weight Loss book are:
- Does Saffron Extract really work?
- What are the probable reason saffron extract work in reducing craving
- Is saffron extract effective for non-compulsive eaters?
- Research findings on saffron extract weight loss
- Other health benefits of saffron extract
- Saffron extract side effects
- Brands of Saffron Extract
- Is saffron extract for everyone who is overweight or obese?
- Healthy meals using saffron extract

In addition, you will also find the following basic information on saffron and saffron extract in this book:
- What is Emotional Eating
- What is saffron?
- Quality standard, Grades and Classification of saffron

Are All Natural Supplements Safe?

Many people have the notion that as long as a substance is natural or labeled as 'natural', it is safe to consume it. While natural food grade substances are normally safe within the scope of 'normal' usage, there could be times when things can get out of the safety zone. I think in some ways, saffron extract fit into this scenario.

Foundational Knowledge

In this book, I also talk about some of the foundational topics such as what saffron is and how saffron is graded and classified, etc. Again, these may be 'common' knowledge to some but many do not know what saffron is. So, I have summarized these basic or background information as appendices of this book. These may not be of interest to everyone who bought this book. But if you are someone who likes to be informed on everything or have a more complete picture of the subject matter, I hope the appendices will serve that purpose for you.

With that, let's dive into this interesting and exciting topic of Saffron Extract Weight Loss.

Jonas Lee

Kuala Lumpur, Malaysia

Chapter 2. Saffron Extract Weight Loss

When **saffron extract** first hit the spotlight on **Dr. Oz** show, it was broadcasted as '**Miracle Appetite Suppressant**'. The central message was the *control of emotional eating* using a commercial brand saffron extract, Satiereal, patented and produced by a company in France, Inoreal Ltd.

The weight loss effects were very convincing as seen on Dr. Oz show, where he had two of his overweight audience to take the supplement for 3 days. One lost 3 lbs while the other 5 lbs. Both participants expressed significant reduction in the urge to snack and reduced appetite. The proposed mechanism is the enhancement effect of saffron extract on serotonin, a hormone that controls the mood and appetite of a person.

Research on Saffron Extract Weight Loss

In performing a literature research, I could find only one clinical trial published in 2010 on weight loss using saffron extract. That study was mentioned in Dr. Oz show involving the Satiereal saffron extract supplement. Another study on mice looking at the effect of saffron on anorexia was published by different researchers in 2011.

Satiereal 1st Clinical Trial

The 1st trial using Satiereal started in 2006 with 16 participants, investigating the efficacy and tolerability of the saffron extract. In other words, they are looking at the beneficial effects and side effects of the supplement.

The trial was conducted with supplemented subjects and a placebo group (the control, without supplementation). After 28 days of supplementation with Satiereal, the outcome of the trials was:
- Decrease in food intake in all supplemented subjects due to feeling of satiety
- Decrease of hunger in all supplemented subjects in the beginning of meal time
- Decrease in meal duration for all supplemented subjects

- Reduction in body weight and fat mass for all supplemented subjects, and
- Reduced desire and pleasure associated to food intake mass for the supplemented subjects

Published Clinical Trial on Saffron Extract Weight Loss Using Satiereal

Later, the researchers (Gout, Bourges and Paineau-Dubreuil) conducted a more elaborate, second clinical study which was subsequently published in Nutrition Research in 2010. The published research paper is entitled *'Satiereal, a Crocus sativus L extract, reduces snacking and increases satiety in a randomized placebo-controlled study of mildly overweight, healthy women'*.

This was a randomized, placebo-controlled, double-blind study, involving 60 healthy and mildly overweight women aged from 25 to 45 years old with BMI of 25 to 28 kg/m². The study was conducted over 8 weeks with the supplemented subjects taking 176.5 mg of the Satiereal saffron extract orally per day.

The number of supplemented subjects was 31 while the placebo group had 29 participants. The study was designed to be homogenous for both groups in terms of age, body weight and snacking frequency. The study looked at various parameters such as body weight, snacking frequency, other anthropometric (body measurements used in physical anthropology) dimensions and vital signs. The last 2 groups of parameters were included to check on tolerability and side effects. There was no restriction placed on calorie or food type.

Results of the Clinical Trial

The results were conclusive and convincing as the Satiereal saffron extract was shown to:

- Reduce snacking and increase satiety significantly in the supplemented women,
- Produce significantly greater weight loss in the supplemented subjects than the control group after the 8 weeks period
- Have no side effects or subject dropout indicated by the stability of other body measurements and vital signs

Conclusion of the Clinical Trial

Based on the results of the trial, the researchers, Gout and coworkers, hypothesized that oral supplementation with Satiereal, a saffron extract, may reduce snacking and enhance satiety through mood improving effect, leading to body weight loss. The researchers also mentioned combining the saffron extract with adequate diet might be a good weight loss program.

Interpretation of the Clinical Trial

Let us summarize the conclusive results of the above clinical trial:

1. Satiereal was able to reduce a person's urge to snack,

2. Satiereal supplementation led to significant weight loss due to reduced food intake, and

3. Satiereal supplementation did not trigger any side effects.

The clinical study had shown the above 3 findings clearly based on the data obtained. The researchers did not claim Satiereal or saffron extract was able to increase production of serotonin.

False Interpretation Misleads People

I am very particular about correct interpretation of research results. This is in part due to the training I received during my days doing graduate research with the intention to publish paper in scientific journal.

Another reason is the rampant incidences of misinterpretation of research data on the internet. False interpretation will mislead people searching for the correct information to make the right decision.

Beware of False Information on the Internet

If you were to do a Google search for the generic term or the brand name, you will likely find 1 to 4 of the top 10 listing on page 1 containing false claims and misinterpretation of the research findings. I have listed some of them below for your reference (without mentioning the sources).

"Satiereal®'s clinically proven formula improves levels of ... serotonin."

"...88.25 mg capsules provide the right amount of safranal and crocin to help regulate serotonergic receptors that induce satiety feelings."

"Just two 88.25 mg capsules of ...Saffron with Satiereal® delivers the active constituents safranal and crocin, shown to modulate certain serotonergic receptors..."

"...saffron extract has the potential to increase mood and serotonin to the brain..."

"… saffron extract has shown saffron to increase the production of serotonin…"

Do not believe in everything you read on the internet!
When you read an article or webpage that claims research studies had shown or proven saffron extract, saffron or Satiereal to be effective in INCREASING the level of serotonin, you can be sure the writer or the website owner does not know his or her topic or is simply making things up out of imagination or creativity. My hunch is those are product pushers.

The study neither claimed nor proved the *increase* of serotonin level due to saffron or Satiereal. The researchers merely HYPOTHESIZED Satiereal likely had an effect in improving the mood of the subject. They did not make that claim. Dr. Oz also did not say the research study made that finding. The animation video he used on his show merely demonstrated to the audience the effect of serotonin on mood and appetite.

Implications and Examination of the Clinical Trial
I will attempt to consolidate the research finding here before we close the chapter. I hope the following

presentation will put things in better perspectives for my readers.

A. Saffron Extract is for Emotional Eaters
A.1. Emotional Eaters

Emotional eaters are persons who reach out for food even though they are not hungry. They have a condition known as **compulsive eating**. The stereotype is quite distinct in that they eat not because of physical hunger but because of some other *emotional or psychological trigger*.

While the behavioral characteristics of emotional eaters are very similar, the underlying cause which makes them devour food compulsively can be drastically different. We will not discuss the root causes of compulsive eating here but I have included a section on this subject in the appendix. If you would like to know a little more about this topic, please refer to Appendix 1.

A.2. Can't Emotional Eaters Put a Rein on Themselves?

No. They can't. That's why they are emotional eaters who consume food by compulsion. They really are at the mercy of their own feeling. It is as though they could not feel they have eaten enough.

The compulsive eating behavior is actually irrational as it is not controllable by reasoning. In other words, it is uncontrollable and the urge is similar to alcoholism and drug addiction. It is like substance abuse. The person's urge overrides the rational capacity.

There are extreme cases where the person literally stuffs himself or herself until they vomit! This sounds funny but it happens in some of the really severe cases. Then the cycle would repeat itself unless they puke themselves to the point of energy drain.

The opposite extreme of emotional eating is anorexia where a person detests the sight of food. Again severe cases of anorexic individuals will literally throw up at the sight of food. The anorexic can die from lack of nutrition and food intake while the emotional eaters literally bloat themselves to overweight and obesity. Both groups of sufferers are incapable of putting a rein on their own behavior.

A.3. Saffron Extract Stops the Sensation of Incessant Need to Snack

The amazing result of saffron extract boils down to its effectiveness in putting a stop to the compulsive behavior of reaching out for food. This is what marvels even the emotional eaters themselves. It's as though the person has regained a newly found control mechanism for their bottomless appetite.

There are a wide range of reactions and experience for those who have been taking saffron extract. Most felt a sense of relief from the constant desire to put food in their mouth. Some did go through a brief period of wavering emotion but the saffron extract fought a winning battle for the person in the end.

A.4. Apparent Weight Loss Resulting From Reduced Food Intake

This is a fairly straight forward and obvious outcome. When you eat less than you normally do, your body will burn any excess fat storage in the body. When you reduce food intake by a large amount, the weight loss will be much greater.

We need to remind ourselves that emotional eaters do consume an irrationally excessive amount of food when they are on binge eating. Therefore, when saffron extract gets into the person and begins to do its job, the food intake reduction can be very significant. That is why we observe a faster and bigger weight loss from them.

In other words, saffron extract is said to have an effect on **compulsive eating behavior**, resulting in subsequent weight loss. Somehow, saffron extract has the ability to stop or reduce a person's cravings or the urge to snack and reach out for food. This reduction in snacking or craving leads to a decrease in food intake, thereby a consequent reduction in body weight.

A.5. Postulated Working Mechanism of Saffron Extract

Based on the results of other scientific studies surrounding serotonin, particularly in the field of depression and mood, it is highly likely that saffron extract has an enhancing effect on serotonin level of the subjects though the above clinical study did not measure the serotonin level in the trial.

Serotonin is a mood regulator

Serotonin is a hormone synthesized in our body. It plays the role of a primary mood neurotransmitter in the brain. A neurotransmitter regulates the signal level between nerve cells. In the case of serotonin, it regulates the transmission of mood signals.

Mood can affect a wide range of behavior, including learning, eating, emotion, sexual behavior, and sleep. Much research has been conducted in the area of depression, which is a mood disorder. Most depression drugs are designed to boost or enhance serotonin level.

Effects of Serotonin Levels

Serotonin level changes with season. Scientists also discovered male and female serotonin systems differ. This is probably the reason why men and women handle stress and anxiety differently.

When serotonin level is high, we feel happy. On the contrary, low level of serotonin will make a person feel depressed. When serotonin level gets higher, it has the effect of sedation. That's why serotonin is related to sleepiness.

Excessively high levels of serotonin will lead to too much nerve cell activity, resulting in serotonin syndrome or serotonin reuptake syndrome, which includes a whole range of symptoms such as dilated pupils, change in blood pressure, rapid heart rate and seizure. When serotonin levels become too low, it can trigger psychiatric condition and may also be the cause of sudden infant death syndrome.

Serotonin – The most Probable Explanation for Saffron Extract Effect on Weight Loss

Serotonin seems to be the most probable explanation for the weight loss effect of saffron extract even without the objective evidence. Abundant research studies on serotonin and mood support the proposed hypothesis of the researchers in the Satiereal study.

The saffron extract may be able to enhance the level of serotonin which leads to a positive change in mood of the subject, accompanied by the reduced desire to snack or reach out for food compulsively. However, there is no direct evidence showing the increase of serotonin due to supplementation of saffron extract.

B. Supplementation Level of Saffron Extract

The Satiereal clinical trial used a daily supplement level of 176.5 mg throughout the 8 weeks period. Unfortunately, the clinical trial used only one level of supplementation. This can raise many concerns for the consumers.

B.1. Why 176.5 mg?

We need to ask the question why this particular recommended intake was used. It would be much more convincing if there is a study that tested the different levels of supplementation on effectiveness and tolerance. Continuing research is necessary if they really believe in their research finding. Having done scientific research in the past, I do understand it is not easy to get funding for continuing research if the researchers are not able to come up with a convincing proposition and justification for the next study.

There really is a whole range of related questions we need answers before this saffron extract can be regarded as a largely safe supplement to consume. Would 200mg work better without any side effects? What would happen if the supplementation continues for 6 months or one year? What would be the level that triggers side effects for most overweight persons?

B.2. Optimal Level of Supplementation

Currently, we have no way of knowing how much serotonin is enhanced, if it did increase the hormone level. This is an important piece of information we must have because we do not want our serotonin to increase to a level where serotonin syndrome kicks in.

B.3. Differences between Male and Female Responses

The study was conducted with female only. Previous research studies on serotonin implied differences of serotonin system between the gender. Assuming saffron extract or Satiereal is able to enhance the level of serotonin, what would be the responsiveness to the supplement between the sexes?

C. Working Mechanism of Saffron Extract

To find out how saffron extract works in the body for losing weight should be the next follow-up study. This is necessary not only for the sake of knowledge but also important for the end users.

Understanding the working mechanism of any substance will provide clues on many aspects, including suitable candidates for taking the supplement, persons who should not be taking the product, etc.

C.1. Is Saffron Extract Able to Enhance Serotonin Level?

This is really an important point to have answers since saffron extract was postulated to enhance or improve the mood of the subjects. This would be related to B.2 and B.3. The study needs to address the changes of serotonin level for different supplementation levels and between male and female.

C.2. What is the Active Ingredient Responsible for Weight Loss?

Saffron contains a huge number of chemical components. Is it crocin, crocetin picrocrocin, safranal or other ingredients responsible for the effect? In order to understand how saffron extract work in the body, we need to know which ingredient is having an effect on the mood of the person. This will be part of understanding the working mechanism of the mood-improving characteristics of the supplement.

Concluding Remarks for Saffron Extract as Weight Loss Supplement

Will the researchers continue with follow-up trials? We have yet to see any further published paper since 2010. I think continuing research in this 'Miracle Appetite Suppressant' is necessary as there are so many issues and questions which must be addressed for long term viability of using this supplement.

Does Saffron Extract Work?
Sure, it does as proven by the clinical studies, but with a lot of precautions and conditions to be considered before one should take it. My view is that the clinical trial published in 2010 was a good start but many aspects of the supplement need to be explored for further understanding and use with confidence.

My reservations in recommending this 'Miracle Appetite Suppressant' to everyone were implied in the above discussion. I will attempt to summarize them here as to why not everyone should be taking the supplement.

- The study was only carried out with a very narrow group of females ONLY who fit a very narrow health and weight profile.

- The level of supplementation was not tested for optimal intake
- We do not know whether male persons will respond just as effectively
- We also do not know whether side effects will be more prevalent in male
- The study was conducted for 8 weeks. We are not sure how long a person can continue taking the supplement without causing any side effects.

There are many other issues I could list that deter me from recommending this supplement. If you do fit in the criteria of their studies, it is probably worth a shot. Otherwise, I would not be comfortable in recommending this supplement though the quality of the brand may be superior.

If you do decide to try out this supplement, please read the chapter on 'side effects' (Chapter 4) before you begin taking it. That's probably the best advice I could give you.

Chapter 3. Other Claimed Health Benefits of Saffron Extract

Other than the recent hype about its weight loss effect, Saffron has been claimed for a myriad of health benefits. Some are based on historical applications while others are based on recent scientific studies. We will take a look at these benefits in this chapter.

List of Saffron Extract Health Benefits
A list of diseases and conditions which saffron has been shown or claimed to be effective is shown below for your reference.

Mood and Emotion-related Conditions
Depression, fright, shock, mental disorders, insomnia

Neurodegenerative or Nerve-related Conditions
Alzheimer's disease, Parkinson's disease, memory, neurasthenia

Related to Digestive System
Digestion, intestinal gas (flatulence), heartburn, dyspepsia

Circulation System or Heart-related Problems
Hardening of the arteries (atherosclerosis), lower blood pressure, improved blood circulation to retina of the eye, induce sweating

Respiratory System Problems
Asthma, cough, whooping cough (pertussis), loosen phlegm (as an expectorant), spitting up blood (hemoptysis), phthisis

Skin Problems
Dry skin, acne, insect bites and stings, better complexion

Related to Pain
Pain, menstrual cramps, premenstrual syndrome (PMS), arthritis, sore throat, hemicrania

Male Problems
Premature ejaculation, aphrodisiac

Other Problems
Colic, edema, prolapse of anus, cancer, apoplexy, liver disorders, splenic disorders, tumors, macula lutea,

infertility, baldness (alopecia), improving weak
eyesight

A. Research-based Health Benefits

A.1. Saffron and Depression

Depression has become a widespread condition and
public health concern today. It is a mood disorder due
to prolonged period of negative emotions such as
sadness, emptiness, guilt, anger, loss, hopelessness,
frustrations, etc.

Depression is a very complex condition where the root
cause can be very variable. Its root cause could be due
to certain life events, medications, infectious diseases,
and psychiatric reasons. As a result, treatment of
depression may require a combination of medical
intervention as well as psychiatric counseling.

Clinical Studies on Saffron Extract for Depression
Other than medical prescription, one of the potential
alternatives is herbal medicine. A group of researchers
from Iran has conducted a series of studies looking at
saffron and depression disorder.

Akhondzadeh and coworkers conducted a 6-week
randomized and double blind clinical trial in 2004,

comparing saffron and imipramine efficacy in treating mild to moderate depression. Imipramine is an antidepressant prescription drug used in treatment of depression. This preliminary study was probably the first clinical trial that showed saffron has therapeutic effect on depression.

In 2005, they did a follow-up study over a 6-week period using double-blind, placebo-controlled and randomized trial. They supplemented the subject with 30 mg of saffron extract per day over the 6 weeks and reported significant alleviation of depression compared to the placebo or control group.

In another preliminary work by Noorbala et al, they found that saffron was as effective as the drug fluoxetine in the treatment of depression. Fluoxetine is another drug used to treat depression but is known for some possible side effects of erectile or sexual dysfunction, anorexia, and asthenia. (Saffron Extract on Sexual Dysfunction is discussed in later section of this chapter)

In 2007, Agha-hosseni et al reported that saffron extract may ease the symptoms of premenstrual symptoms including depression in double blind placebo controlled trial.

Conclusion on Saffron Extract and Depression
Clinical studies indicate that saffron extract provides promising effect on treatment of depression. Saffron extract holds great potential in replacing some of the drugs used in depression treatment.

It is interesting to note that only 30 mg per day is required to produce improvement in depression studies compared to 176.5 mg per day in the case of weight loss trial.

A.2. Saffron Extract on Neurodegenerative Disorders
Neurodegenerative disorders are marked by progressive dysfunction or death of nerve cells. Examples of neurodegenerative diseases are Parkinson's, Alzheimer's and Huntington's diseases.

To date, there is no known medical cure for neurodegenerative diseases. Medical treatment involves medications which lessen the symptoms, or slow down the progress of the disease.

Research studies searching for the cure for neurodegenerative diseases have been ongoing for decades. Unfortunately, none has been able to provide promising cure of these debilitating illnesses.

Research on Saffron Extract on Learning and Memory

Some of the most significant symptoms of neurodegenerative diseases include progressive loss of memory and the ability to learn. Severe cases of neurodegenerative diseases can result in patients losing the basic skills of life. It is as though they have to re-learn how to feed themselves, how to take bath, etc.

As a result, many studies zero in on the cognitive aspects and/or memory functions of the patient. Though not a cure for the root cause, the studies will help improves management of the neurodegenerative disorders.

In 2000 Abe and Saito looked at the effect of crocin, a component of saffron extract, on learning and long term signal transmission between nerve cells. They pointed out that saffron extract or its active constituents, crocetin and crocin, could be useful as a treatment for neurodegenerative disorders accompanying memory impairment.

In 2011 Papandreou and coworkers studied the effect of saffron on cognitive and memory functions of mice. Their results showed that saffron-treated mice exhibited significant improvement in learning and memory. The study also showed that significant cognitive enhancement due to saffron in mice was more closely related to the antioxidant reinforcement.

Another study conducted in the same year by researchers Ghadrdoost et al looked at chronic stress induced learning and memory deficits in rats. They found that saffron and crocin (active constituent of saffron) were able to prevent the impairment of learning and memory as well as the chronic stress induced oxidative stress damage to the hippocampus.

In 2012 another group of researchers led by Hosseinzadeh performed experiments in rats which suggested that saffron extract and crocin improved spatial cognitive abilities following chronic cerebral hypoperfusion (inadequate supply of blood to the brain, can lead to brain damage and cell death). They argued that the effects may be related to the antioxidant effects of these compounds.

Conclusion on Saffron Extract on Neurodegenerative Disorders

Despite all the technical jargons in the above research studies, the results by different group of researchers essentially showed promising potential of saffron, particularly its active component crocin, in reversing learning and memory damages which are typical consequences of neurodegenerative disorders. The studies also demonstrated that crocin possesses antioxidant power that can help prevent damages in learning and memory capacity.

However, the next stage of research would be to conduct human clinical trials before saffron can be safely used on human to treat neurodegenerative disorders.

A.3. Saffron Extract on Anorexia.

An interesting study published in 2011 was to look at the effects of saffron extract on stress-induced anorexia in rats. Halataei and his team of researchers looked at how saffron, safranal and crocin impact the food intake, weight gain and anorexic duration in mice.

Their results showed that saffron extract and crocin both reduced the stress-induced anorexia in the mice, but the safranal (a component of saffron) was not able to relieve the mice from the anorexia.

The studies basically showed that different components of the saffron extract may have different or opposite effects on anorexia or weight gain.

A.4. Saffron Extract on Cancer and Tumor
It appears there is more and more evidence and work done on the cancer-fighting properties of saffron extract.

In 1991 Nair and his coworkers experimented with mice and showed the anticancer property of saffron extract. In a review summary by Nair in 1995, he said his laboratory work on saffron indicated carotenoid-like actions on cancerous growths such as carcinoma, sarcoma and leukemia. Another series of experiments were carried out by Abdullaev and his coworkers, looking at saffron extract effects on antitumor and chemopreventive properties.

Without going into the details of a whole bunch of published papers, we summarize here the important findings regarding the effects of saffron extract on cancer:

- Laboratory studies indicate saffron possesses anticancer effects
- Feeding mice with saffron extract inhibited both the initiation and the promotion of cancer, thus preventing the formation of soft tissue sarcomas (malignant tumors that originate in the soft tissues of the body).
- Saffron extract was able to extend the life span of mice which had undergone chemotherapy with cisplatin (a chemotherapy drug used to treat cancer of the testicles, bladder, ovaries, or lung), which has the side effects of causing kidney damage
- Saffron extract was also able to extend the life span of mice with tumors
- Crocin, a carotenoid in saffron, was shown to slow down colon cancer growth in female rats

and increased survival time of female rats, but had no significant effects in male rats.

- Saffron was shown to inhibit synthesis of nucleic acid, DNA or RNA, in cancer cells
- Saffron has a promising antioxidant property indicated by the increased level of reduced glutathione and glutathione-related enzymes within the cells
- Saffron may be a potential chemotherapeutic agent in lung cancer treatment indicated by the ability of saffron to induce apoptosis (programmed cell death in cancer cells)

A.5. Saffron Extract on Sexual Dysfunctions

Saffron has also been claimed to be a strong aphrodisiac herb. Let's take a look at some of the studies done in this area.

Depression-related Sexual Dysfunction

The antidepressant drug fluoxetine is known to induce sexual dysfunction in patients taking the drug. As a result, some studies were done to determine the effect of saffron on fluoxetine-induced sexual dysfunction.

In 2012 Modabbernia et al conducted a 4-week randomized double-blind placebo-controlled study. They studied 36 married male patients who were treated and stabilized with fluoxetine and who also had subjective complaints of sexual impairment. The supplemented patients were given 15mg saffron twice a day for 4 weeks. Having 30 patients completed the study their findings showed that saffron resulted in significantly greater improvement in erectile function. Their study also indicated that 60% of the saffron supplemented patients and 7% of the placebo group achieved normal erectile function. This study indicated that saffron is a tolerable and efficacious treatment for fluoxetine-related erectile dysfunction.

In another study Kashani et al looked at 38 women who were also treated and stabilized with fluoxetine. The supplemented group were given 30 mg of saffron daily for 4 weeks. Their results demonstrated that saffron may safely and effectively improve some of the fluoxetine-induced sexual problems including arousal, lubrication, and pain.

Erectile Dysfunction

Shamsa et al studied the effect of saffron on male erectile dysfunction in 2009. The study followed 20 male patients with erectile dysfunction for 10 days. They took 200mg of saffron in tablet form each morning. Tests were taken prior to and at the end of the 10-day study. Results showed positive effect on sexual functions indicated by increased number and duration of erectile events.

In 2010 Safarinejad and coworkers did a larger scale study with 346 men, aged from 38 to 54 years old, with erectile dysfunction. They used a daily supplementation level of 30 mg saffron, taken twice a day. Their results indicated that saffron had no beneficial effect on men with erectile dysfunction.

Conclusion on Saffron Extract on Sexual Dysfunctions

It appears that saffron extract may or may not have an effect on sexual dysfunction. In the published studies different persons responded differently. One major reason may be the supplementation level for varying severity of sexual dysfunction. More detailed studies are needed before a more concrete recommendation for saffron extract to be used to treat sexual dysfunction or as aphrodisiac.

A.6. Saffron Extract on Premenstrual Syndrome (PMS)

Premenstrual syndrome or PMS are common female health problems during their reproductive age. Also, premenstrual dysphoric disorder or PMDD, a severe subtype of PMS, affects 3–8% of women of reproductive age. The symptoms are often marked by severe behavioral and mood changes.

In 2008 Agha-Hosseini and coworkers from Tehran University of Medical Sciences studied the effects of Saffron on premenstrual syndrome. They selected 50 women, aged from 20 to 45 years old and who had premenstrual syndrome symptoms such as bloating, cramp, fatigue and irritability for at least 6 months. They randomly split the 50 women into 2 groups, one group taking placebo capsule while the other group taking 15 mg saffron capsule twice a day. The study was conducted over 2 menstrual cycles. Their study indicated that 75% of the women taking saffron had at least a 50% less in PMS symptoms while only 8% from the placebo group had that. The study demonstrated saffron may well be an alternative treatment for PMS.

In 2011 an interesting study by Fukui and coworkers investigated the effect of saffron odor on symptoms typically experienced by women, such as premenstrual syndrome (PMS), dysmenorrhea (menstrual pain) and irregular menstruation. Their results demonstrated that saffron odor had some effects in the treatment of PMS, dysmenorrhea and irregular menstruation. This is the first study that suggests saffron odor may be effective in treating menstrual distress.

A.7. Closing

It appears saffron extract has a lot of potential for medicinal and therapeutic purposes. However, our understanding of saffron properties in medicine and therapy is still very limited as more studies need to be done before we understand this gift of nature.

Schmidt et al gave a comprehensive review on the phytotherapy uses of saffron. Indeed, much research studies are yet to be conducted to fully exploit the potential of saffron. Some of the studies on antidepressant properties have been performed in laboratory as well as in clinical trials. However, cancer studies using saffron require clinical trials before it can be used on cancer patients.

The potential of saffron for treatment makes sense because saffron contains abundant volatile and non-volatile components. Many of the components or constituents are carotenoids which are known for promoting health.

Consuming Medical Herb for Prolonged Period

I hope you have a reasonably good appreciation of the medical potential of saffron from this chapter. With that understanding in mind, we need to have some answers or indications on:

- ✓ *'Is it safe to consume a medicinal herb in large quantity for prolonged period?'*
- ✓ *'Are there any negative reactions from the body on consuming saffron extract?'*
- ✓ *'Is it safe for pregnant lady?'*

With that, let's proceed to the next chapter on side effects.

Chapter 4. Saffron Extract Side Effects

A woman went to her doctor for a follow-up visit after the doctor had prescribed testosterone (a male hormone) for her. She was a little worried about some of the side effects she was experiencing. "Doctor, the hormones you've been giving me have really helped, but I'm afraid that you're giving me too much. I've started growing hair in places that I've never grown hair before." The doctor reassured her, "A little hair growth is a perfectly normal side effect of testosterone. Just where has this hair appeared?"

"On my testicles, which is something else I want to talk to you about...," replied the lady.

Conflicting Information on Side Effects

If you tried to search for information on saffron safety or side effects, you will be confused as to who has the right information. Some state no side effects while others indicate the opposite. This makes it very frustrating and confusing for those who really want to know the answers before they feel it's safe to consume saffron extract.

Saffron Extract Side Effects

You will find both extreme when it comes to saffron extract side effects. Studies had been done to determine the body's tolerance for different level of saffron.

No or Slight Adverse Effects at 400 mg Saffron?

Modaghegh et al evaluated short-term safety and tolerance of saffron tablets in healthy adults. They conducted a double-blind, placebo-controlled trial with 3 groups of subjects. Each group consisted of 5 males and 5 females. Group 1 was the control while groups 2 and 3 were supplemented with 200 and 400 mg saffron tablets respectively for 7 days. Their results showed that at 400 mg supplementation level, blood pressure was reduced and some minor changes in blood-related characteristics such as red blood cells, hemoglobin, hematocrit and platelets. However, the researchers concluded that the changes were still within normal ranges and bore no clinical importance.

Mohamadpour and coworkers also investigated the short-term safety of crocin, a constituent of saffron, in tablet form. Their results indicated no adverse effects. However, crocin did decrease amylase, mixed white blood cells and PTT in healthy volunteers after one month. They concluded crocin a relatively safe for healthy persons at the given doses within the trial period.

Adverse Effects with 30 mg Saffron?
However, clinical trials on depression using daily dosages of 30 mg saffron showed no statistically significant adverse effects between supplemented subjects and placebo group, but adverse effects such as nausea, vomiting, and headache were reported.

Side Effects with High Doses
For culinary usage, the amount of saffron used is generally less than 5 g. Ingesting 5 g of saffron was reported to cause severe purpura (which is the appearance of red or purple discolorations on the skin), thrombocytopenia (a condition with abnormally low amount of platelets), and severe bleeding.

At a dosage of 10 g saffron, it acts like an *abortifacient*, which is a substance that induces abortion. When saffron dosage gets to excessively high level of 20 g, it becomes lethal.

Possible Responses

Though there are no studies indicating many of the potential side effects or responses, you will see them commonly mentioned and discussed in many of the medical websites. They are included here for your perusal.

Some possible mild symptoms from taking saffron extract may include anxiety, dryness of the mouth, giddiness, nausea, headache, loss of or reduced appetite, and allergic reactions.

Possible poisoning may include vomiting, dizziness, blood in diarrhea, yellowish skin, yellowish eyes and yellowish mucous membrane, nose bleed, numbness and bleeding lips and eyelids.

Possible Risks for Pregnant Women And Women Who Are Breast-Feeding
As mentioned above large intake of saffron at 10g will have the effect of an abortifacient. At this level of saffron, it may trigger contraction of the uterus, which could lead to miscarriage. There is no recorded incidence of saffron extract supplement causing side effects on women who are breast-feeding, but some medical websites advise it is safer for them to refrain

from intake of the saffron extract.

Chapter 5. Brands of Saffron Extract

Overview of Saffron Extract Supplement on Amazon
I feel that the book will not be complete without a list of saffron brands in the market place. Please note that this is not a recommended list. I have not tried any of the brands as I am not into weight loss myself. And I am not endorsing any brand in particular.

The overview is more for the convenience of viewing the different brands in one place. Unfortunately, I could not include a summary table here as it will not be viewable in Kindle. The order is based on the first 10 saffron extract products listed in Amazon and a summary of some pertinent information here. I hope this overview gives you some idea of the different brands. (Price may change over time)

1. Saffron Extract by Genetic Solutions

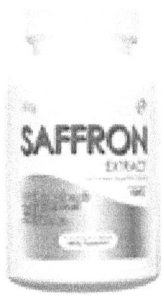

Price = $27.85 & FREE Shipping (List Price = $49.95; Save = $22.10 (44%))

Size = 90 Veggie Capsules (88.5mg), 2 capsules per day for 45 days

Made in = USA

Average Customer Review = 3.5 Star (5 Star=124; 4 Star=50; 3 Star=24; 2 Star=23; 1 Star=53)

No. Customer Reviews = 274

Some customer Reviews:

5 star, "Killer Combination!" February 4, 2013. Benjamin

5 star, "Not hungry!" June 3, 2013. A. Bruzzi

2 Star, "DOES NOT WORK!!!!!" July 6, 2013. B. Tatman

2 Star," My appetite was not suppressed" June 29, 2013. Christina Barbosa.

2. Optimized Saffron with Satiereal by Life Extension

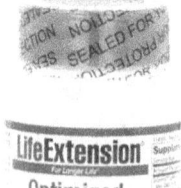
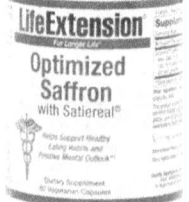

Price = $16.99 (List Price = $39.20; Save = $22.21 (57%))

Size = 60 Vegetarian Capsules (88.25 mg), 2 capsules per day for 30 days

Made by = Satiereal for Quality Supplements and Vitamins, Inc. Ft, Lauderdale, Florida

Average Customer Review = 3 Star (5 Star=30; 4 Star=15; 3 Star=14; 2 Star=15; 1 Star=25)

No. Customer Reviews = 99

Some customer Reviews:

5 Star, "willpower in a bottle" November 13, 2011. S. Lawless

5 Star, "Subtle but WOW!" July 27, 2012. Pat Ellingson

3 Star, "For Weight Loss?" July 29, 2013. desertsyl

2 Star, "Not what I had hoped for." June 18, 2013. Cinjes "Ca" (CA)

3. Pure Saffron Extract Appetite Suppressant by Source Health Labs

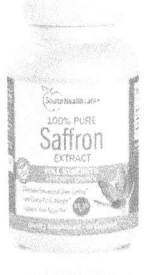

Price = $19.77 & FREE Shipping on orders over $25
(List Price = $39.99; Save = $20.22 (51%))
Size = 60 Capsules (88.25 mg), 2 capsules per day for 30 days
Made in = USA
Average Customer Review = 4.5 Star (5 Star=11; 4 Star=0; 3 Star=1; 2 Star=1; 1 Star=1)
No. Customer Reviews = 14
Some customer Reviews:
5 Star, "It Really Works!!!!!" July 20, 2013. R. Thomas "Gina" (St. Louis, MO)
5 Star, "Easy to Take" April 8, 2013. Gloria (PLANT CITY, FLORIDA, United States)
3 Star, "Too Subtle of Results" July 24, 2013. S. Chapman
1 Star, "Didn't do anything" July 15, 2013. C. Erickson (Detroit, MI)

4. ReBody Hunger Caps with Satiereal Saffron Extract by Re-Body

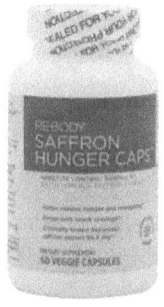

Price = $16.25 ($0.27 / count) & FREE Shipping on orders over $25 (List Price = $29.99; Save = $13.74 (46%))

Size = 60 Veggie Capsules (88.5 mg), 2 capsules per day for 30 days

Made in = USA

Average Customer Review = 3 Star (5 Star=85; 4 Star=27; 3 Star=24; 2 Star=34; 1 Star=63)

No. Customer Reviews = 233

Some customer Reviews:

5 Star, "Great appetite suppressant with NO SIDE EFFECTS" September 13, 2012. BookChick

4 Star, "Works great to control hunger!" July 21, 2012. Deborah Gilmore

2 Star, "Didn't work" June 3, 2013. Stephanie Hartley

1 Star, "Nothing" September 19, 2012. SHargis (California)

5. Saffron Pure l 88.5mg l 90 Count l Two Bottle Pack! By Saffron Pure

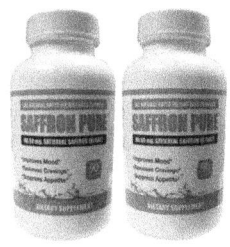

Price = $29.95 ($14.98 / Item) (List Price = $59.90; Save = $29.95 (50%))

Size = 90 Veggie Capsules (88.5 mg) per bottle, 2 capsules per day for 45 days (2 bottles=90-day supply)

Made in = USA

Average Customer Review = 3 Star (5 Star=9; 4 Star=3; 3 Star=4; 2 Star=12; 1 Star=8)

No. Customer Reviews = 36

Some customer Reviews:

5 Star, "Love it!" May 3, 2013. Kristine Schroder "Ticker" (Grand Island, NE)

4 Star, "Best price found!" February 23, 2013. Renee C. Burton

2 Star, "Heartburn!" February 26, 2013. D. Hill (Kaysville, UT USA)

1 Star, "Did not do a thing" March 31, 2013. William Witkowski

6. 100% Pure Premium Saffron Extract by Holistic Solutions

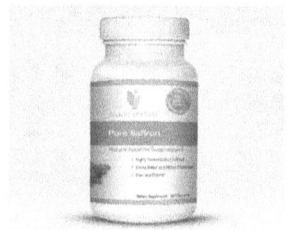

Price = $18.99 & FREE Shipping on orders over $25
(List Price = $49.00; Save = $30.01 (61%))

Size = 60 Capsules (88.25 mg) per bottle, 2 capsules per day for 30 days

Made in = USA

Average Customer Review = 4 Star (5 Star=4; 4 Star=1; 3 Star=0; 2 Star=0; 1 Star=1)

No. Customer Reviews = 6

Some customer Reviews:

5 Star, "So Happy" August 18, 2013. Carol Knight

5 Star, "Pure and Clean" August 18, 2013. Julius Johnson (USA)

1 Star, "Snake oil in disguise?" August 18, 2013. J. R. Goldsberry (Dover DE)

7. Only Natural - Standardized Saffron Extract Made With Saffr'Activ, 88 mg, 30 veggie caps by Only Natural

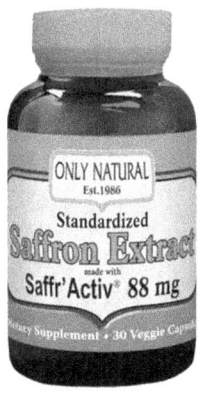

Price = $11.22 ($3.74 / 10 Items) & FREE Shipping on orders over $25 (List Price = $24.95; Save = $13.73 (55%))

Size = 30 Capsules (88 mg) per bottle

Made in = Not Available on Amazon

Average Customer Review = 4 Star (5 Star=5; 4 Star=5; 3 Star=3; 2 Star=0; 1 Star=1)

No. Customer Reviews = 14

Some customer Reviews:

5 Star, "unexpected benefit" March 5, 2013. PAD

4 Star, "It's a good product." March 13, 2013. Jennifer

3 Star, "Couldn't tell" October 17, 2012. Sam

1 Star, "nothing" June 18, 2013. Andrea L.

8. Saffron Extract 50 Count by Bio Nutrition

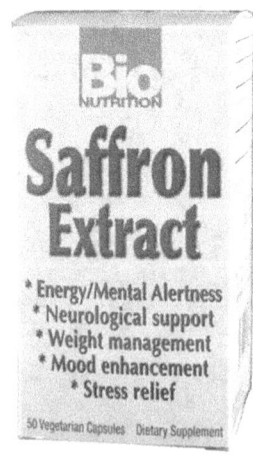

Price = $9.49 ($3.30 / oz) & FREE Shipping on orders over $25 (List Price = $15.99; Save = $6.50 (41%))

Size = 50 Vegetarian Capsules (88.5 mg), 1 capsule per meal, 3 per day

Made in = Not mentioned on Amazon

Average Customer Review = 4 Star (5 Star=5; 4 Star=1; 3 Star=0; 2 Star=2; 1 Star=0)

No. Customer Reviews = 8

Some customer Reviews:

5 Star, "curb appetite" February 12, 2013. Rossie Dallas

5 Star, "Helps me stay focused!" May 24, 2013. Adam Spade "Adam Spade" (Indiana)

2 Star, "Not working" April 30, 2013. Goldie "Goldie" (NJ)

9. Best Naturals, Appetite Control, 100% Pure Premium Satiereal Saffron Extract by Best Naturals

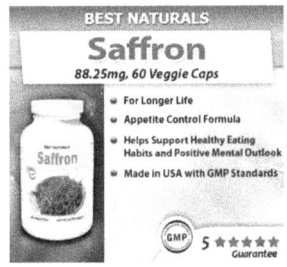

Price = $15.99 & FREE Shipping on orders over $25 (List Price = $31.99; Save = $16.00 (50%))

Size = 120 Veggie Caps (88 mg)

Made in = USA

Average Customer Review = 3 Star (5 Star=16; 4 Star=11; 3 Star=4; 2 Star=8; 1 Star=18)

No. Customer Reviews = 57

Some customer Reviews:

5 Star, "Keeps me feeling full & satisfied" May 25, 2012. MSCKaren (Florida Beach)

4 Star, "Good stuff" May 28, 2013. Sandra Chapman

1 Star, "not as advertised" April 25, 2013. SEC

10. Saffron Extract- Appetite Suppressant - 100% Pure Premium Saffron Extract - 88mg - 120 Capsules - 120 Servings Per Bottle by Hydra Health Saffron Extract

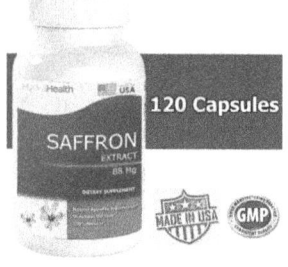

Price = $16.49 & FREE Shipping on orders over $25 (List Price = $49.95; Save = $33.46 (67%))

Size = 120 Veggie Caps (88 mg)

Made in = USA

Average Customer Review = 3.5 Star (5 Star=7; 4 Star=2; 3 Star=4; 2 Star=5; 1 Star=2)

No. Customer Reviews = 20

Some customer Reviews:

5 Star, "Saffron extract really suppresses appetite" April 7, 2013. artistined

4 Star, "ok - no miracle pill" May 1, 2013. bg

2 Star, "Don't waste money!" July 3, 2013. Amanda O'Connor

1 Star, "Does not work" July 2, 2013. rosemary

Chapter 6. Healthy Meals Using Saffron Recipes

"Let food be thy medicine and medicine be thy food" -
Hippocrates

Food is always the Best Remedy

The father of medicine, Hippocrates, said it best through his philosophy of looking into food for sustaining our health. There is no doubt that food should always be our permanent, long term strategy and lifestyle to maintaining and sustaining long lasting health.

In line of using food as the best health keeper, I have selected various recipes which use saffron in their preparation. Please take note of the sources of recipes, where you may find the original recipe and also other recipes of interest to your taste.

1. Saffron Basmati Rice (Sunny Anderson)

Source of recipe
=http://www.foodnetwork.com/recipes/sunny-anderson/saffron-basmati-rice-recipe/index.html

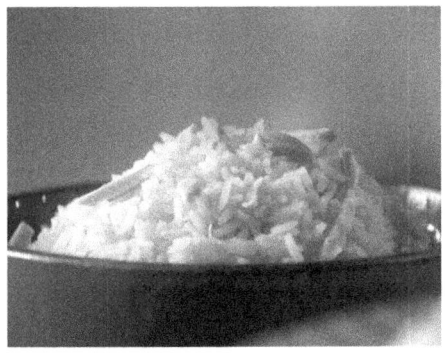

Total Time: 30 min (Prep Time=10 min, Inactive Time=5 min, Cook Time=15 min)

Ingredients: (for 4 to 6 servings)
2 cups basmati rice, 1 tablespoon olive oil, 1 clove garlic, smashed
3 to 4 threads saffron, Pinch of cayenne pepper, 3 to 3 1/2 cups chicken stock, 1/4 cup almond slivers, toasted
1 teaspoon lemon zest, Salt and freshly ground black pepper

Directions:
Rinse the rice in a colander under cold water until it runs clear, picking out any little pieces of grit or debris. Shake off the excess water. Heat a pot over medium heat, and then add the rice, oil, garlic, saffron and cayenne pepper. Stir and toast the rice until the cayenne and saffron are fragrant, about 4 minutes.

Shake the pot to level out the rice, and then add the chicken stock to fill about 1/2-inch over the rice. Bring to a boil, and then lower to a simmer and cover to cook for 15 minutes. Remove from the heat and let the rice stand another 5 minutes, covered. Fluff with a fork. Stir in the almond slivers and lemon zest, season with salt and pepper and serve.

2. Iberian-Style Sausage & Chicken Ragù (Eating Well)

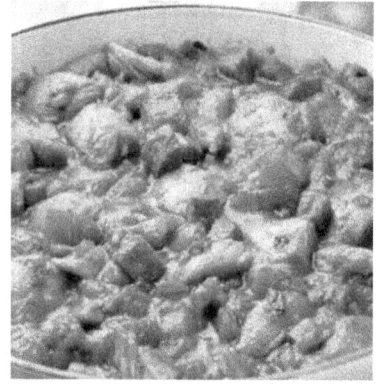

Source of recipe =
http://www.eatingwell.com/recipes/iberian_sausage_chicken_ragu.html

Total Time =2 hours 10 minutes (Active Time=1 hour)
Ingredients :(for 16 servings, about 8 cups)
1 tablespoon extra-virgin olive oil; 8 ounces linguisa (Portuguese-style sausage) or Spanish-style chorizo,

diced; 3 cups chopped onion; 2 tablespoons finely chopped garlic; 2 tablespoons Pimentón de la Vera (see Note); 2 pounds boneless, skinless chicken thighs, trimmed and cut into 1-inch chunks; 1/2 teaspoon kosher salt; Freshly ground pepper to taste; 3 cups white wine; 4 cups diced seeded tomatoes or canned diced tomatoes; 2 cups reduced-sodium chicken broth; 1/4 cup chopped flat-leaf parsley; 1 generous pinch saffron threads (see Note);

Directions:

Heat oil in a large pot or Dutch oven over medium heat and add sausage. Cook, stirring occasionally, until the edges begin to color, 5 to 10 minutes. Add onion and garlic. Cover and cook for 10 minutes, stirring occasionally, until the onion is quite soft.

Sprinkle Pimentón de la Vera over the onion mixture; stir to coat. Cook for 1 minute. Add chicken, salt and pepper; stir to coat. Cook, stirring, for 5 minutes. Add wine and increase heat to high; cook until the wine is reduced by about a third, about 8 minutes.

Stir in tomatoes, broth, parsley and saffron; reduce heat to maintain a simmer and cook, uncovered, until the chicken is tender and the sauce is beginning to thicken, 1 to 1 1/4 hours. Season with more pepper, if desired.

Tips: Make Ahead Tip: Refrigerate in an airtight container for up to 5 days or freeze for up to 3 months.

Notes: Spain is known for its superb paprika called Pimentón de la Vera, which has a smoky flavor. Look for it in well-stocked supermarkets, gourmet-food shops or online at tienda.com.

The dried stigma from Crocus sativus, saffron adds flavor and golden color to a variety of Middle Eastern, African and European foods. Find it in the spice section of supermarkets, gourmet shops or at tienda.com. It will keep in an airtight container for several years.

Nutrition: 185 calories; 7 g fat (2 g sat , 2 g mono); 38 mg cholesterol; 7 g carbohydrates; 16 g protein; 1 g fiber; 230 mg sodium; 312 mg potassium.

3. Baked Spanish risotto (Silvana Franco)

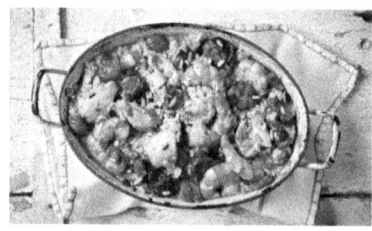

Source of recipe = http://www.bbc.co.uk/food/recipes/bakedspanishrisotto_702 41

Preparation Time=30 min (Cooking Time=30 min to 1 hour)

Ingredients: (4 servings)
250g/9oz cherry tomatoes; 1 red onion, finely chopped; 2 garlic cloves, finely chopped;
2 tbsp olive oil; 300g/10oz risotto rice; 4 chicken thigh fillets, halved; 200g/7oz chorizo, thickly sliced; 2 tsp chopped fresh rosemary; 1 litre/1¾ pints hot chicken stock; pinch of saffron strands; 8 large, raw prawns; salt and freshly ground black pepper

Directions:
1. Preheat the oven to 220C/425F/Gas 7. Place the cherry tomatoes in a roasting tin and sprinkle over the red onion, garlic and olive oil. Roast for 20 minutes until the tomatoes are softened.
2. Stir in the rice, chicken, chorizo, rosemary, chicken stock, saffron and some salt and pepper, mixing well together. Return to the oven for 20 minutes.
3. Stir in the prawns and return to the oven for a further 10 minutes until the rice is tender and the chicken is cooked through.

4. Grilled Saffron Rack of Lamb (Samin Nosrat)

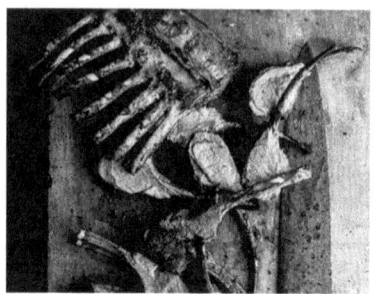

Source of recipe =
http://www.epicurious.com/recipes/food/views/Grilled-Saffron-Rack-of-Lamb-51169130

Note: The lamb needs to marinate overnight, so be sure to start 1 day ahead

Ingredients: (6 servings)

2 racks of lamb (3-3 1/2 pounds total), rib bones frenched; Kosher salt, freshly ground pepper; 2 garlic cloves, crushed; 1 cup plain 2% fat Greek yogurt; 2 tablespoons olive oil; 1 teaspoon finely grated lemon zest; 1/2 teaspoon saffron threads, finely crumbled.

Directions:

Season lamb with salt and pepper and place each rack of lamb in a large resealable plastic bag. Whisk garlic, yogurt, oil, lemon zest, and saffron in a small bowl and divide between bags. Seal bags, pressing out excess air; turn to coat. Refrigerate lamb overnight.

Prepare grill for medium-high, indirect heat. (For a charcoal grill, bank coals on 1 side of grill; for a gas grill, leave 1 burner turned off.) Remove lamb from marinade and wipe off excess. Place lamb over direct heat and cook, turning and moving to cooler part of grill as needed to avoid flare-ups, until browned all over, 8-10 minutes.

Move lamb to cooler part of grill. Cover grill and cook lamb, turning occasionally, until an instant-read thermometer inserted into the center registers 125° for medium-rare, about 15 minutes longer.

Let lamb rest 10 minutes. Cut into individual chops.

5. Steamed Mussels with Wine and Saffron (Martha Stewart's Cooking School)

Source of recipe =
http://www.marthastewart.com/951456/steamed-mussels-wine-and-saffron

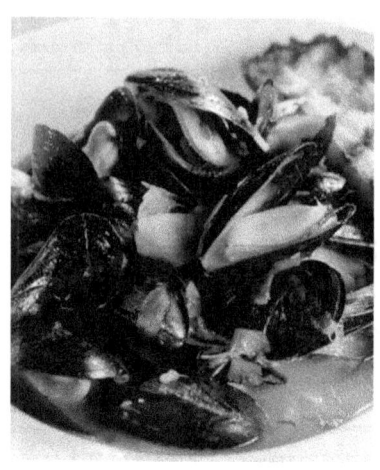

Ingredients:

3 pounds fresh mussels; 1 large pinch saffron (about 30 threads); 3/4 cup dry white wine; 2 tablespoons unsalted butter; 2 medium shallots, thinly sliced (about 1/2 cup); 2 garlic cloves, thinly sliced; Coarse salt and freshly ground pepper; 2 medium tomatoes, coarsely chopped (about 2 cups); 1/4 cup coarsely chopped fresh flat leaf parsley.

Directions:

1. Holding mussels under cool running water, scrub with a stiff sponge or vegetable brush, then debeard: grip the tough fibers extending from the shell and pull to remove. Discard beards.

2. Steep saffron in wine for 10 minutes. (Saffron is soluble in water, not fat, so it won't release its color or flavor if added directly to the butter.) Meanwhile, melt butter over medium-high heat in a shallow stockpot. Once it's foamy, add shallots, garlic, and 1/2 teaspoon salt. Cook until shallots are transparent and garlic is soft, about 3 minutes, stirring every so often to keep garlic from scorching. Pour in wine and saffron, then add tomatoes and return to a simmer, stirring once or twice.

3. Add mussels and cover tightly. Cook until all mussels open, about 6 minutes, stirring once about halfway through. Discard any unopened mussels. If using wild mussels, strain broth through a cheesecloth-lined sieve to remove any sand, if necessary. Taste the broth and season with salt and pepper.

4. Sprinkle with parsley before ladling mussels and broth into bowls.

6. Kashmiri Chicken, Cardamom and Saffron Pilau: Spiced Indian Rice (French Tart)

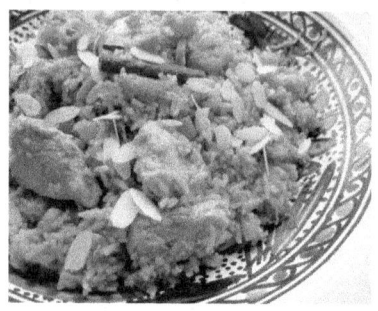

Total Time =1 h 30 min (Prep Time = 30min; Cook Time = 1 h)

Ingredients:

1 lb white basmati rice; 2 tablespoons oil; 2 onions, peeled and diced; 4 garlic cloves, peeled and crushed; 1 inch fresh gingerroot, peeled and finely diced; 2 teaspoons cumin seeds; 1 1/2 lbs boneless chicken or 1 1/2 lbs boneless chicken breasts, cubed; 1 teaspoon saffron strand; 1/2 pint boiling water; 6 cardamom pods, bruised; 4 tablespoons chopped fresh mint; 2 teaspoons garam masala; 1 cinnamon stick; 8 ounces skinned and chopped tomatoes or 8 ounces tinned chopped tomatoes; 2 ounces sultanas; salt; pepper; 2 ounces blanched almonds, toasted.

Directions:

1. Rinse the basmati rice several times in cold water and drain in a colander - leave to dry.
2. Heat half of the oil (1 tablespoon) in a large pan and add half of the onion (1 onion), the garlic, ginger and cumin seeds. Fry them over a gentle heat for about 5 minutes.
3. Add the chicken pieces and brown them - turning them regularly to achieve a good colour all over.
4. Add the saffron, boiling water, cardamom pods, mint, garam masala and cinnamon stick. Bring it all to the boil and then cover, reduce the heat and simmer for 25 to 30 minutes, until the chicken is tender.
5. Transfer all the contents to a bowl and rinse out the pan.
6. Add the remaining oil and onion to the pan and fry until the onion is lightly coloured. Add the rice and stir it well, cook for about 2 to 3 minutes until the rice is opaque.
7. Add the chicken mixture, tomatoes and sultanas - then season to taste with salt and pepper. Stir gently, then shake the pan to level the ingredients.

8. Add sufficient boiling water to come about 3/4" above the rice mixture. Cover with a tight fitting lid and cook gently over a low heat for 20 to 25 minutes, until the rice is tender and the liquid has all been absorbed.
9. Discard the cinnamon stick and transfer to a warm serving dish, sprinkle with the toasted almonds and serve immediately.

7. Saffron Biscotti (Stockholm's famed Vete-Katten bakery)

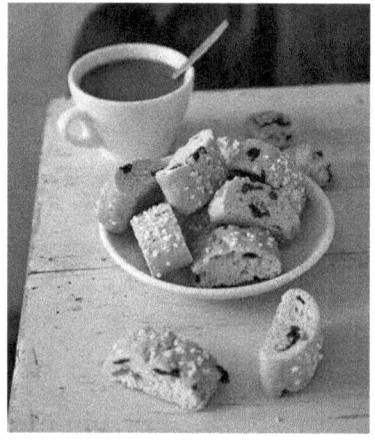

Source of recipe =
http://www.saveur.com/article/Recipes/Saffron-Biscotti

Ingredients: (Makes about 40 cookies)
3 cups flour; 2 tsp. baking powder; 1/2 tsp. kosher salt; 1 cup sugar; 4 tbsp. unsalted butter, softened;   1 tbsp.

orange zest; 1 tsp. saffron, lightly crushed; 2 eggs;
1/4 cup milk; 3.5 oz. dark chocolate, chopped; Pearl
sugar, for garnish.

Directions:

1. Heat oven to 325°. Whisk together flour, baking
   powder, and salt in a medium bowl; set aside. In
   a large bowl, using a handheld mixer on
   medium speed, beat together sugar, butter,
   orange zest, and saffron until pale and fluffy, 1–2
   minutes. Add the eggs one at a time, beating
   well after each addition; add milk and mix until
   combined. Reduce mixer speed to low and add
   dry ingredients in 3 additions; mix until just
   combined. Mix in chocolate, then transfer dough
   to a work surface.

2. Quarter dough, transfer each quarter to a
   parchment paper–lined baking sheet, and form
   each into a 12" x 1" flattened log; sprinkle each
   log with 1 tbsp. pearl sugar and refrigerate for 20
   minutes. Bake 1 sheet at a time until lightly
   browned around edges, 30–35 minutes. Transfer
   baking sheet to a wire rack and let cool for 15
   minutes; repeat with remaining dough logs.

3. Reduce oven temperature to 300°. Transfer each
   log to a cutting board and, using a serrated

knife, slice the logs into 1"-thick slices. Return slices to the baking sheet, cut sides up and spaced evenly apart, and bake 1 sheet at a time until light brown and dry, 15–20 minutes; transfer to a wire rack to let cool completely before serving.

8. Syrian Chicken with Ginger, Lemon & Saffron (Karen Martini)

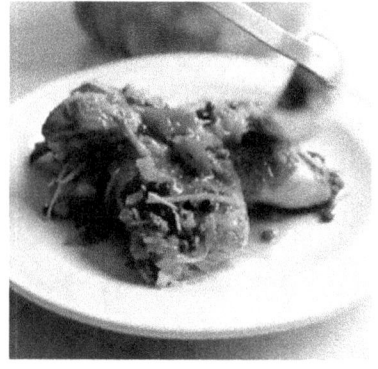

Source of recipe = http://karenmartini.com/cook/recipes/syrian-chicken-ginger-lemon-saffron

Total Time =1 h (Prep Time = 20min)
Ingredients:
2 teaspoons salt; 2 teaspoons ground cumin; 2 teaspoons ground cinnamon; 1 teaspoon ground black pepper; 1 teaspoon ground turmeric; 1.4–1.6 kg

chicken, cut into 8 pieces; 100 ml extra virgin olive oil; 2 brown onions, thickly sliced; 100 grams ginger, cut into matchsticks; 5 cloves garlic, peeled and crushed with the side of a knife; 2 small red chillies, split; 2 tomatoes, coarsely chopped; 2 pinches saffron threads; ½ teaspoon cumin seeds; 5 sprigs thyme, leaves only; 1 lemon, juiced and zested; 2 tablespoons honey; 100 grams currants; 2 tablespoons vegetable stock powder; ½ bunch coriander, leaves only couscous or rice, to serve

Directions:

1. Combine the salt, cumin, cinnamon, pepper and turmeric in a large plastic bag. Add the chicken pieces and shake to coat.

2. Heat the olive oil in a large heavy-based saucepan over high heat. Add the chicken and brown on all sides. Remove from the pan and set aside. Add the onion, ginger, garlic and chilli to the pan and cook for 3 minutes, adding a little more oil, if necessary. Add the tomatoes, saffron, cumin seeds and thyme and cook for 2 minutes.

3. Return the chicken to the pan and add the lemon juice and zest, honey, currants, stock powder and enough water to just cover the chicken.

4. Cover with a lid and simmer over medium heat for 10 minutes. Uncover and simmer for 10-15 minutes or until the chicken is tender and cooked through, and the sauce is slightly reduced.

5. Stir in the coriander and serve with couscous or rice.

9. Saffron Halwa Recipe (rida naz)

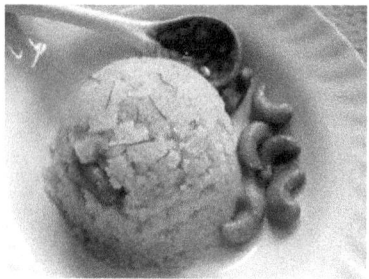

Source of recipe =
http://karachifoods.com/saffron_halwa_rid2763

Ingredients:

RIce flour 2cups; Sugar 2 cups; Clarified Butter 300 gram; Green Cardamoms 4; Dried Milk 1 cup; Fresh Cream 1 cup; Almond (fried) 50 gram; Screwpine 1 tbsp; Saffron ½ tsp.

Directions:

Heat oil clarified butter in a wok; add rice flour and fry; remove from flame.

Add saffron, sugar, cardamoms, dried milk, crem and screwpine; mis well and put on dum.remove from flame when clarified butter separtes

Dish out halwa, garnish with almonds

10. Seafood Stew in Saffron Broth (Kitchen Daily)

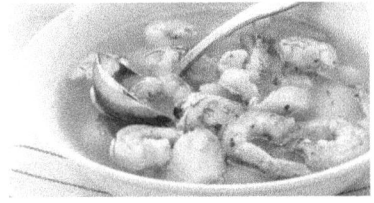

Source of recipe = http://www.kitchendaily.com/recipe/seafood-stew-saffron-broth

Ingredients: (For 4 servings)
6 cup reduced-sodium chicken broth; 2 tsp saffron threads; 2 tsp Italian seasoning blend (preferably salt-free); 8 oz medium shrimp, peeled and deveined; 8 oz cod, cubed

Directions:
Combine the broth, saffron, and seasoning blend in a large saucepan over medium-high heat. Bring to a simmer.

Add the shrimp and cod and simmer for 3 to 5 minutes, until the seafood is opaque and cooked through. Season to taste with salt and freshly ground black pepper before serving.

Chapter 7. Is Saffron Extract Weight Loss For You?

Saffron extract weight loss as discussed in chapter 2 works well with female emotional eaters who are overweight. Saffron extract is able to reduce the urge to snack or eat compulsively. This may be due to its effect on serotonin which controls the mood of the person.

Too Many Unknowns

I personally feel there is too much unknown in this so called 'Miracle Appetite Suppressant'. In addition, the parameters used in the clinical study were narrow and limited to be interpreted as suitable for all persons who are emotional eaters.

Problem of Supplementation Level

Other than the issue of dosage or supplementation level, the subjects were only female. This opens a lot of unknown whether or not the dosage used is applicable to the male emotional eaters, as previous research studies implied differences between male and female serotonin system.

No Universal Supplementation Level

Looking at the research studies of saffron on a wide range of body conditions and illness, you will notice there is no universal dosage used on different conditions. This further complicates and confuses the issue of appropriate level of supplementation.

Saffron is Medicine

After you have read this book, you probably get the impression that saffron is such an amazing substance given to us by nature. The potential it holds for many aspects of our body and health is beyond our current status of understanding. I hope you also realize from the discussion in this book that saffron possesses medical property, though their details and mechanism remain unclear.

Saffron is also a Spice

Some may argue that for thousands of years saffron has been used as food. So, it should not have any adverse effects on our body. I tend to think that because saffron as spice is mixed, prepared or cooked with other food, it may not behave like the pure extract taken without any mixing and cooking. Again, we have no answers.

Conclusion

A short term use of saffron extract for weight loss is probably fairly safe and sound, if you keep watch of any potential responses mentioned in chapter 4. I strongly disagree using a substance with drug like properties to control one's emotion. Honestly, do you want to rely on a drug-like substance to help curb your eating habit? If a person feels strongly that his or her eating behavior or habit is uncontrollable, I think it's better to seek treatment rather than zap oneself with a substance with so many unknowns.

I also think that the health properties of saffron are undeniable. Perhaps, one might want to incorporate saffron into our diet more often, though it might not be a regular part of one's cultural dishes. After all, let food be your medicine and build up our health with the right food.

I hope you have enjoyed reading this book as much as I have enjoyed writing it. I deeply appreciate if you could return to Amazon and post your honest review on this book. Thanking you in advance.

Take good care and be of great health!

Jonas Lee

Apendix 1. Emotional Eating

Emotional and Compulsive Eating

Emotional eating is not an action to satisfy hunger. Though the person may not feel hungry, he or she still has the urge or habit to reach out for food. This is typical behavior of a person with habitual cravings and compulsive overeating. The sensation of wanting to eat in emotional eater is not driven by physical hunger. The cravings and the irrational urge to eat is developed as a result of other life, emotional or psychological events.

Typically, what will happen is the emotional eater will not feel satiated even though he or she has consumed beyond his or her normal capacity. In other words, the person will go on with episodes of binge eating. When this pattern becomes too frequent, it really is an illness known as binge-eating disorder. So, an emotional eater tends to be overweight or obese.

Emotional Hunger Versus Physical Hunger

Most of us have probably experienced emotional eating in ourselves one time or another. When we do that occasionally to satisfy our emotion, it's not a problem. When the frequency of emotional eating picks up, that's when a bigger problem is looming within.

One important sign of emotional eating is we eat to satisfy an emotion. The emotion can be sadness, loneliness, happiness, self-pity, anxiety, stress, etc. In other words, it can be any emotion.

When we reward ourselves with food for achieving something significant, that's fine because not too many of us experience big achievements daily. But when we reward our stomach due to happiness and if we are happy most days, then that spells trouble.

Many people who have just broken up in a relationship tend to develop emotional eating. Somehow the sensation of eating is linked to the sensation of satiety for people in such emotional state. The act of eating becomes a way to fill the void left behind from a broken relationship or other traumatic experience.

Apendix 2. What is Saffron?

Saffron Comes from a Flower

Saffron is the name of a spice obtained from a flower known as Saffron Crocus, also scientifically called Crocus sativus. The crocus is a member of a family of flowering plants known as iris. The iris is a perennial grown from corm.

The crocus normally bears flowers in the winter, spring or autumn. They are grown for their beautiful bulbous flowers. Most people have seen one or more form of crocus flowers as they are commonly used for their ornamental value. Some of the common crocus flowers are Dutch crocus, Saffron crocus, Autumn crocus, Spring Crocus, and Winter crocus.

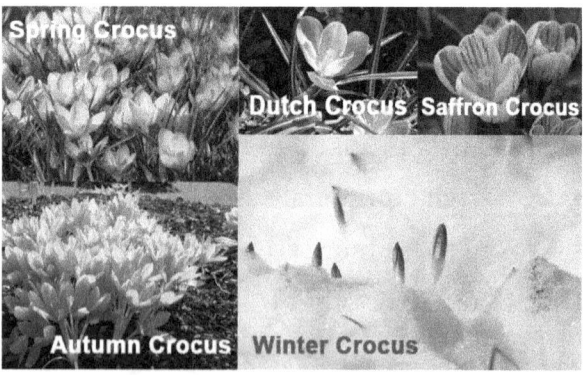

(Sources of photos - *Dutch crocus*: **http://commons.wikimedia.org/wiki/File:Crocus_1.jpg**); *Saffron*

crocus:
http://commons.wikimedia.org/wiki/File:RNK_1556_safran.jpg;
Autumn crocus:
http://www.flickr.com/photos/aardvarkoffnord/1422448022/;
Spring crocus: http://pixabay.com/p-3944/?no_redirect; *Winter
crocus*:
http://www.flickr.com/photos/vasile23/8606299884/sizes/o/in/phot
ostream/)

Origin of Saffron

Saffron original came from the wild species known as
Crocus cartwrightianus. Saffron crocus is considered to
be a mutant of its wild species. Over the course of
domestication and cultivation, the cultivated saffron
has undergone long history of cultivar selection to
consist of long stigmas. This is logical as the stigmas are
the major parts of the flower harvested though the
petals are also used.

It appears that saffron has been cultivated for more
than 3,000 years.

Saffron is a Spice

Saffron is most famous for its use in cooking as spice.
The stigma of the saffron crocus is harvested and dried
before it can be used as a spice (refer to diagram
below).

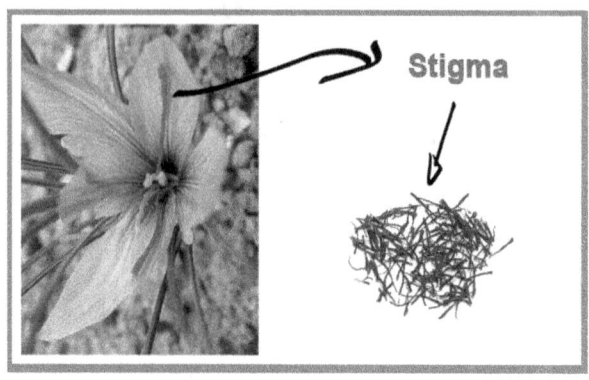

(Source of saffron flower :
http://commons.wikimedia.org/wiki/File:Crocus_sativus_01_by_Li
ne1.JPG)

As you can imagine, it requires a lot of human labor to pluck out the stigmas from the saffron flower before they are dried. According to Bas Deo (ref. 1) of Crop & Food Research from New Zealand, Saffron is the world's most expensive spice.

Saffron Uses in Cooking and Other Purposes
Saffron has been used as a seasoning, fragrance, dye, and medicine for more than 3,000 years. Saffron has been used over the centuries as a natural coloring and aromatic in food, pastries and drinks. Saffron is used extensively in many cultures, including Persian, European, North African, Indian, Spanish, Arab, Turkish, Moroccan, and Asian cuisines.

Experts said the aroma of saffron is like that of honey, intermingled with a bit of grassy, hay-like, and metallic notes. Saffron has a bitter taste. Saffron stigmas are red but when it is wet it becomes a yellow-orange dye or color. With these characteristics saffron is used in baked foods, rice, cheeses, confectionaries, curries, liquors, meat dishes, soups, macaronis, and even ice creams.

One of the most common functions of saffron is to make the rice yellow. This can be seen in risotto Milanese, where the flavor of saffron marks the characteristic of Italian rice dishes.

Saffron goes well with fish and seafood. Saffron is a key ingredient of Persian chicken and beef kabob, Spanish paella, Mexican fiambre, Arabic lamb and chicken, Azerbaijani pakhlava, and Indian pilafs, desserts and sauces as well as French bouillabaisse.

Nutritional Value of Saffron
The following tables are taken from the National Nutrient Database of the United States Department of Agriculture.

Nutrient	Unit	1 Value per 100.0g	# of Data Points	Std. Error	1.0 tbsp 2.1g	1.0 tsp 0.7g
Proximates						
Water	g	11.90	111	0.247	0.25	0.08
Energy	kcal	310	--	--	7	2
Energy	kJ	1298	--	--	27	9
Protein	g	11.43	12	0.684	0.24	0.08
Total lipid (fat)	g	5.85	17	0.737	0.12	0.04
Ash	g	5.45	103	0.084	0.11	0.04
Carbohydrate, by difference	g	65.37	--	--	1.37	0.46
Fiber, total dietary	g	3.9	--	--	0.1	0.0
Minerals						
Calcium, Ca	mg	111	1	--	2	1
Iron, Fe	mg	11.10	1	--	0.23	0.08
Magnesium, Mg	mg	264	--	--	6	2
Phosphorus, P	mg	252	1	--	5	2
Potassium, K	mg	1724	3	251.548	36	12
Sodium, Na	mg	148	2	--	3	1
Zinc, Zn	mg	1.09	--	--	0.02	0.01
Copper, Cu	mg	0.328	--	--	0.007	0.002
Manganese, Mn	mg	28.408	--	--	0.597	0.199
Selenium, Se	µg	5.6	--	--	0.1	0.0
Vitamins						
Vitamin C, total ascorbic acid	mg	80.8	--	--	1.7	0.6
Thiamin	mg	0.115	--	--	0.002	0.001
Riboflavin	mg	0.267	--	--	0.006	0.002
Niacin	mg	1.460	--	--	0.031	0.010
Vitamin B-6 [1]	mg	1.010	2	--	0.021	0.007
Folate, total	µg	93	--	--	2	1
Folic acid	µg	0	--	--	0	0
Folate, food	µg	93	--	--	2	1
Folate, DFE	µg	93	--	--	2	1
Vitamin B-12	µg	0.00	--	--	0.00	0.00
Vitamin A, RAE	µg	27	--	--	1	0
Retinol	µg	0	--	--	0	0
Vitamin A, IU	IU	530	--	--	11	4
Vitamin D (D2 + D3)	µg	0.0	--	--	0.0	0.0
Vitamin D	IU	0	--	--	0	0

Lipids						
Fatty acids, total saturated	g	1.586	--	--	0.033	0.011
4:0	g	0.000	--	--	0.000	0.000
6:0	g	0.000	--	--	0.000	0.000
8:0	g	0.000	--	--	0.000	0.000
10:0	g	0.000	--	--	0.000	0.000
12:0	g	0.000	--	--	0.000	0.000
14:0	g	0.006	--	--	0.000	0.000
16:0	g	1.157	--	--	0.024	0.008
18:0	g	0.247	--	--	0.005	0.002
Fatty acids, total monounsaturated	g	0.429	--	--	0.009	0.003
16:1 undifferentiated	g	0.003	--	--	0.000	0.000
18:1 undifferentiated	g	0.390	--	--	0.008	0.003
20:1	g	0.006	--	--	0.000	0.000
22:1 undifferentiated	g	0.000	--	--	0.000	0.000
Fatty acids, total polyunsaturated	g	2.067	--	--	0.043	0.014
18:2 undifferentiated	g	0.754	--	--	0.016	0.005
18:3 undifferentiated	g	1.242	--	--	0.026	0.009
18:4	g	0.000	--	--	0.000	0.000
20:4 undifferentiated	g	0.013	--	--	0.000	0.000
20:5 n-3 (EPA)	g	0.000	--	--	0.000	0.000
22:5 n-3 (DPA)	g	0.006	--	--	0.000	0.000
22:6 n-3 (DHA)	g	0.000	--	--	0.000	0.000
Cholesterol	mg	0	--	--	0	0

Let's take a summary view of the above information. A quick glance tells us that saffron is fairly rich in nutritional value as it consists of a wide spectrum of minerals and vitamins. The values in the 3rd column are based on 100g of saffron. No one in their right mind would consume 100g of saffron. Even the values in the last column, which is for 1 teaspoon, are rarely used. Most recipes recommend anywhere from a pinch of the saffron powder, up to a few grams.

Apendix 3. Saffron Grades & Classification

Normally, the higher the price, the higher will be the quality of saffron. Because saffron is such a high priced commodity, there are incidences where the product is mixed with inferior supplies or outright counterfeit product.

The ISO Standard for Saffron Quality Control
The saffron industry has developed specific criteria to grade and classify the quality of saffron. Today, saffron quality is regulated by the international ISO/TS 3632 standard, which sets in stone a system of quality control. It consists of 2 parts, namely Part 1 the specification (ISO 3632-1:2011) and Part 2 the test methods (ISO 3632-2:2010). The latest version is now ISO/TS 3632-1:2011, which has replaced the previous version of ISO/TS 3632-2:2003.

Without going into the specifics of the criteria, the quality measures according to ISO/TS 3632 include 3 essential characteristics:
1. Crocin concentration,

2. Picrocrocin level, and
3. Safranal level.

1. Crocin Concentration

Crocin is the substance that gives saffron its color, the color of the stigma. It can also be found in the flowers of plants from the coffee family (ref. a). Crocin is a carotenoid with a deep red color and crystallizes at room temperature with a melting point of 186 degree Celsius. It will dissolve in water giving the solution an orange color.

As a carotenoid, crocin has strong antioxidant properties. Research studies indicate that crocin showed promising potential in inhibiting the formation as well as accumulation of substance known as amyloid β-peptide (Aβ) fibrils in the brain of Alzheimer's patients (ref. f). This particular substance has been known to be caused by oxidation. As a result, crocin from saffron may be used in treating Alzheimer's because of its antioxidation property.

The crocin concentration in any saffron product is determined by using what is known as spectrophotometry. We learn in basic science that different colors absorb different amount of light. In other words, they measure the absorbance difference between samples or products. The higher the absorbance, the stronger or darker the color, hence the higher the concentration of a color.

According to ISO standard, different crocin concentrations are assigned different grades as shown in the table below.

Grade	I	II	III	IV
Absorbance	> 190	150 - 190	110 - 150	80 - 110

Based on the above criteria set by ISO 3632, a saffron sample with an absorbance of 200 is considered Grade I, which is the finest quality saffron. Any absorbance from 80 - 110 is deemed to be of poorest quality saffron. If the absorbance falls below 80, a saffron will have no grade at all.

So, if you are comparing different batches of saffron, you can easily tell by the differences in their redness. Grade I saffron should have the deepest red, while Grade III will have darker red than Grade IV.

2. Picrocrocin Level

Picrocrocin is the component that gives saffron its bitter taste. It is the flavoring component of saffron. Picrocrocin is also measured using spectrophotometry. Absorbance of crocin is measured at a wavelength of 440nm while picrocrocin absorbance is measured at 257nm.

ISO 3632 for picrocrocin test is shown in the table below.

Grade	I	II	III	IV
Absorbance	80	70	70	70

Notice that Grade II to Grade IV saffron should have an absorbance of 70 while Grade I saffron is 80.

3. Safranal Level

Safranal is the component that renders the aroma to saffron. This is the substance which gives the odor property of saffron. Again, absorbance of safranal is measured using spectrophotometry at a wavelength of 330nm.

ISO 3632 for safranal test is shown in the table below.

Grade	I	II	III	IV
Absorbance	20 - 50	20 - 50	20 - 50	20 - 50

Based on the above criteria of ISO for saffron, we notice that crocin concentration is the major factor that determines whether or not the saffron is of the finest quality. Therefore, visual inspection of saffron batches should give a good indication of the quality of the products.

References

Chapter 2

Gout B, Bourges C, Paineau-Dubreuil S. Satiereal, a Crocus sativus L extract, reduces snacking and increases satiety in a randomized placebo-controlled study of mildly overweight, healthy women. Nutr Res. 2010 May;30(5):305-13

Chapter 3

Akhondzadeh S, Fallah-Pour H, Afkham K, Jamshidi AH, Khalighi-Cigaroudi F. Comparison of Crocus sativus L. and imipramine in the treatment of mild to moderate depression: A pilot double-blind randomized trial. BMC Complement Altern Med. 2004; 4: 12.

Akhondzadeh S, Tahmacebi-Pour N, Noorbala AA, Amini H, Fallah-Pour H, Jamshidi AH, Khani M. Crocus sativus L. in the treatment of mild to moderate depression: a double-blind, randomized and placebo-controlled trial. Phytother Res. 2005; 19: 148-51.

Noorbala AA, Akhondzadeh S, Tahmacebi-Pour N, Jamshidi AH. Hydroalcoholic extract

of Crocus sativus L. versus fluoxetine in the treatment of mild to moderate depression: a

double-blind, randomized pilot trial. J. Ethnopharmacol. 2005; 97: 281 - 4.

Akhondzadeh Basti A, Moshiri E, Noorbala AA, Jamshidi AH, Abbasi SH, Akhondzadeh

S. Comparison of petal of Crocus sativus L. and fluoxetine in the treatment of depressed outpatients: a pilot double-blind randomized trial. Prog. Neuropsychopharmacol Biol. Psychiatry 2007; 31: 439 - 42.

Abe K, Saito H. Effects of saffron extract and its constituent crocin on learning behaviour and long-term potentiation. Phytother Res. 2000 May;14(3):149-52.

Papandreou MA, Kanakis CD, Polissiou MG, Efthimiopoulos S, Cordopatis P, Margarity M, Lamari FN. (2006). "Inhibitory activity on amyloid-beta aggregation and antioxidant properties of Crocus sativus stigmas extract and its crocin constituents". J Agric Food Chem. 2006 54 (23): 8762–8.

Papandreou MA, Tsachaki M, Efthimiopoulos S, Cordopatis P, Lamari FN, Margarity M. Memory enhancing effects of saffron in aged mice are correlated with antioxidant protection. Behav Brain Res. 2011 Jun 1;219(2):197-204.

Ghadrdoost B, Vafaei AA, Rashidy-Pour A, Hajisoltani R, Bandegi AR, Motamedi F, Haghighi S, Sameni HR, Pahlvan S. Protective effects of saffron extract and its active constituent crocin against oxidative stress and spatial learning and memory deficits induced by chronic stress in rats. Eur J Pharmacol. 2011 Sep 30;667(1-3):222-9.

Hosseinzadeh H, Sadeghnia HR, Ghaeni FA, Motamedshariaty VS, Mohajeri SA. Effects of saffron (Crocus sativus L.) and its active constituent, crocin, on recognition and spatial memory after chronic cerebral hypoperfusion in rats. Phytother Res. 2012 Mar;26(3):381-6.

Halataei BA, Khosravi M, Arbabian S, Sahraei H, Golmanesh L, Zardooz H, Jalili C, Ghoshooni H. Saffron (Crocus sativus) aqueous extract and its constituent crocin reduces stress-induced anorexia in mice. Phytother Res. 2011 Dec;25(12):1833-8.

Nair SC, Pannikar B, Panikkar KR. Antitumour activity of saffron (Crocus sativus). Cancer Lett. 1991 May 1;57(2):109-14.

Nair SC, Kurumboor SK, Hasegawa JH. Saffron chemoprevention in biology and medicine: a review. Cancer Biother. 1995 Winter;10(4):257-64.

Nair SC, Salomi MJ, Pannikar. B, Pannikar KR. Modulatory effects of the extracts of saffron and Nigela sativa against cisplatinum induced toxicity in mice. Journal of Ethnopharmacology, 31:75-83, 1991(a).

Nair SC, Salomi MJ, Varghese CD, Pannikar B, Pannikar KR. Effect of saffron on thymocyte proliferation, intracellular gluthathione levels and its antitumor activity. BioFactors 1992 4(1): 51-54.

Abdullaev FI, Frenkel, G.D. Effect of saffron on cell colony formation and cellular nucleic acid and protein synthesis. BioFactors 1992 3(3): 201-204.

Abdullaev FI, Frenkel G.D. The effect of saffron on intracellular DNA, RNA and protein synthesis in malignant and non-malignant human cells. BioFactors 1992 4(1): 43-45.

Abdullaev, F. Cancer chemopreventive and tumoricidal properties of saffron (Crocus sativus L.). Exp Biology and Medicine 2002 227(1): 20-25.

Abdullaev FI, Riveron-Negrete L, Cabalerro-Ortega H, Hernandez JM, Perez-Lopez I, Pereda-Miranda R, Espinosa-Aguirre JJ. Use of in vitro assays to assess the antigenotoxic and cytotoxic effects of saffron (Crocus sativus L.) Toxicology In Vitro. 2003 17: 731-736.

Samarghandian S, Tavakkol Afshari J, Davoodi S. Suppression of pulmonary tumor promotion and induction of apoptosis by Crocus sativus L. extraction. Appl Biochem Biotechnol. 2011 May;164(2):238-47.

El Daly ES. Protective effect of cysteine and vitamin E, Crocus sativus and Nigella sativa extracts on cisplatin-induced toxicity in rats. Journal de Pharmacie de Belgique. 1998 53(2): 93-95.

Escribano , Alonso GL, Coca-Prados M, and Fernandez JA. Crocin, safranal and picrocrocin from saffron (Crocus sativus L,) inhibit growth of human cancer cells in vitro. Cancer Letters 1996 100:23-30.

Garcia-Olmo DC, Riese HH, Escribano J, Ontañon J, Fernandez JA, Atienzar M, Garcia-Olmo D. Effects of long-term treatment of colon adenocarcinoma with crocin, a carotenoid from saffron (Crocus sativus L.): an experimental study in the rats. Nutrition and Cancer 1999 35(2): 120-126.

Riverón-Negrete L, et al. The combination of natural and synthetic agents: a new pharmacological approach in cancer chemoprevention. Procedures of the Western Pharmacology Society 2002 45:74-75.

Tarantilis PA, Morjani H, Polissiou M, and Manfait M. Inhibition of growth and induction of differentiation promyclocytic leukemia (HL-60) by carotenoids from Crocus sativus L. Anticancer Res 1994 14: 1913-1918.

Schmidt M, Betti G, Hensel A. Saffron in phytotherapy: pharmacology and clinical uses. Wien Med Wochenschr. 2007;157(13-14):315-9.

Shamsa A, Hosseinzadeh H, Molaei M, Shakeri MT, Rajabi O. Evaluation of Crocus sativus L. (saffron) on male erectile dysfunction: a pilot study. Phytomedicine. 2009 Aug;16(8):690-3

Safarinejad MR, Shafiei N, Safarinejad S. An open label, randomized, fixed-dose, crossover study comparing efficacy and safety of sildenafil citrate and saffron (Crocus sativus Linn.) for treating erectile dysfunction in men naïve to treatment. Int J Impot Res. 2010 Jul-Aug;22(4):240-50

Modabbernia A, Sohrabi H, Nasehi AA, Raisi F, Saroukhani S, Jamshidi A, Tabrizi M, Ashrafi M, Akhondzadeh S. Effect of saffron on fluoxetine-induced sexual impairment in men: randomized double-blind placebo-controlled trial. Psychopharmacology (Berl). 2012 Oct;223(4):381-8.

Kashani L, Raisi F, Saroukhani S, Sohrabi H, Modabbernia A, Nasehi AA, Jamshidi A, Ashrafi M, Mansouri P, Ghaeli P, Akhondzadeh S. Saffron for treatment of fluoxetine-induced sexual dysfunction in women: Randomized double-blind placebo-controlled study. Hum Psychopharmacol Clin Exp. 2012;28(1):54-60.

Agha-Hosseini M, Kashani L, Aleyaseen A, Ghoreishi A, Rahmanpour H, Zarrinara AR, Akhondzadeh S. Crocus sativus L. (saffron) in the treatment of premenstrual syndrome: a double-blind, randomised and placebo-controlled trial. BJOG. 2008 Mar;115(4):515-9.

Fukui H, Toyoshima K, Komaki R. Psychological and neuroendocrinological effects of odor of saffron (Crocus sativus). Phytomedicine. 2011 Jun 15;18(8-9):726-30.

Chapter 4

Modaghegh MH, Shahabian M, Esmaeili HA, Rajbai O, Hosseinzadeh H. Safety evaluation of saffron (Crocus sativus) tablets in healthy volunteers. Phytomedicine. 2008 Dec;15(12):1032-7.

Mohamadpour AH, Ayati Z, Parizadeh MR, Rajbai O, Hosseinzadeh H. Safety Evaluation of Crocin (a constituent of saffron) Tablets in Healthy Volunteers. Iran J Basic Med Sci. 2013 Jan;16(1):39-46.

Appendices

Deo, B. (2003), "Growing Saffron—The World's Most Expensive Spice", Crop and Food Research (New Zealand Institute for Crop and Food Research) (20), archived from the original on 27 December 2005, retrieved 10 January 2006

Nutrient data for 02037, Spices, saffron. USDA National Nutrient Database (United States Department of Agriculture).

Dr. Duke's Phytochemical and Ethnobotanical Databases. [Online Database] 05 August 2013. http://www.ars-grin.gov/duke/

About The Author

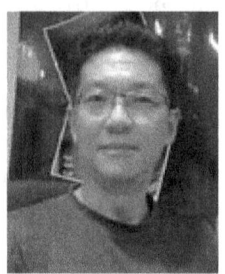

Jonas Lee

Jonas Lee, born in Tawau, Sabah, Malaysia, obtained his Bachelor of Science and Master of Science degrees from the University of Saskatchewan, Canada. Upon his graduation, he started working in the Health industry until today. His career in the health sector has ignited his passion for natural therapy as well as functional foods and supplements.

Jonas has been and is a writer and editor for many health websites for the past decade. Now, he is devoting his time to distill his thoughts and experience on health and treatments onto writings which are suitable for people without the medical or scientific background..

Though Jonas is not a doctor, people from all over the world has written to him through his health websites for opinion and consultation. Jonas walks his talk. His knowledge on a wide range of health topics is more than just filling some space on the internet. He shares his health insights and experience with his family and friends, and friends of friends. He only shares from what he knows is good and speaks what he understands as not advisable. If he is not sure, he will tell you he needs to look into that further.

If you have any questions or comments? Please email him at jonas@healthtips,org.

More from This Author

Coconut Oil Weight Loss - Healthy Long Lasting Fat Loss Without Starving [Kindle Edition]

Link: http://www.amazon.com/dp/B00E1EV97Y

Weight Loss Coconut Oil was his first book, which can be obtained here or click on the book cover below.

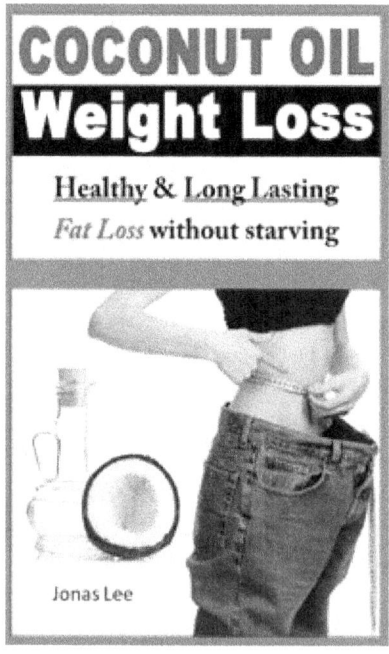

Coconut oil weight loss is about healthy weight loss and healthy fat loss! If you are skeptical about whether coconut oil can really help you lose weight, please read on. I don't blame you for your skepticism as you have probably based your conclusion on some shady articles you had read on the internet.

The author is deeply disturbed by health blog writers, including some doctors and nutritionists, who made irresponsible statements about coconut oil.

If you have come across statements that hinted, implied or outright slammed coconut oil as bad because it is a saturated fat, then the people who made those statements were either too lazy to learn about saturated oils or too hurried to finish some article deadlines and not bother to differentiate the types of saturated fats!

In this eBook the author sets out to present his arguments based on studies and logical interpretation on how and why coconut oil can and will contribute to healthy weight loss. Some of the benefits from reading this eBook are:

• Why should some individuals lose weight while others should not even consider weight loss
• How do you determine you should consider losing some weight

- Know the dangers of quick weight loss
- True weight loss
- How does our body lose weight
- What really is coconut oil
- What are the differences between short-chain, medium-chain, and long-chain fatty acids
- Is coconut oil fattening
- Why are vegetable oils fattening
- Does coconut oil increase your metabolism
- Why isn't coconut oil not stored as fats
- How to take coconut oil
- How much coconut oil should you take
- Why are scientists breeding polyunsaturated fat producing oil crop to produce more saturated fat

Learn about Coconut Oil Weight Loss and more.

A Request From the heart of... Jonas

Once again my heartfelt appreciation for purchasing and reading this book.

I sincerely hope you have benefited from this book, one way or another. Should you have any queries, please write to me at **Jonas@healthtips.org** and I will do my best to answer them. If you have enjoyed this book, I really appreciate if you could return to Amazon and drop a review. Thanking you in advance.

All the best of health,
Jonas
Kuala Lumpur, Malaysia